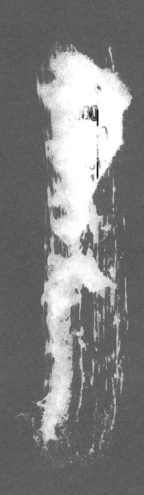

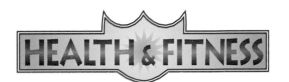

HOW DO
DRINK AND
DRUGS
AFFECT ME?

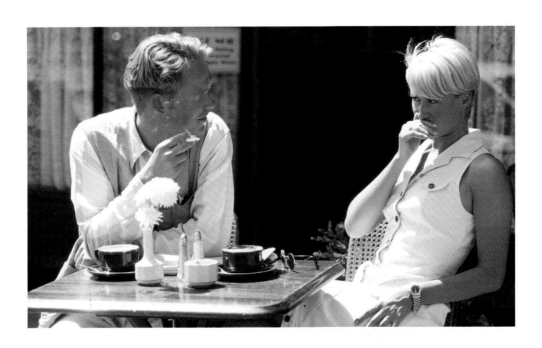

Emma Haughton

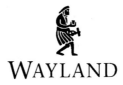

WAYLAND

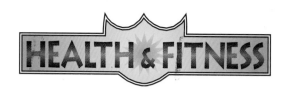

HEALTH & FITNESS

HOW DOES ADOLESCENCE AFFECT ME?
HOW DO DRINK AND DRUGS AFFECT ME?
HOW DOES EXERCISE AFFECT ME?
HOW DOES MY DIET AFFECT ME?

Produced for Wayland Publishers Limited by
Roger Coote Publishing
Gissing's Farm
Fressingfield
Suffolk IP21 5SH
England

Designer: Victoria Webb
Editor: Alex Edmonds
Illustrations: Michael Posen

First published in 1999 by Wayland Publishers Limited
61 Western Road, Hove, East Sussex BN3 1JD

British Library Cataloguing in Publication Data
Haughton, Emma
  How do drink and drugs affect me? – (Health and fitness)
  1. Alcohol – Physiological effect – Juvenile literature
  2. Drugs - Physiological effect – Juvenile literature
  I. Title
  615.7'8

ISBN 0 7502 2571 8

Printed and bound in Italy
by G. Canale & C.S.p.A., Turin

All Wayland books encourage children to read and help them improve their literacy.

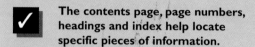 The contents page, page numbers, headings and index help locate specific pieces of information.

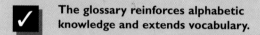 The glossary reinforces alphabetic knowledge and extends vocabulary.

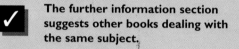 The further information section suggests other books dealing with the same subject.

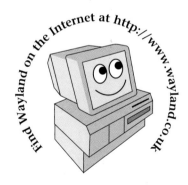

find Wayland on the Internet at http://www.wayland.co.uk

Picture acknowledgements:
Digital Stock *cover band* bottom; Digital Vision 42; Image Bank 4 (Rod Westwood), 10 (David de Lossy), 11 (David de Lossy), 20 (Gabriel Covian), 22 (Bokelberg), 24 (Nicholas Russell), 28 (Color Day), 31 top (Color Day), 32 (Steve McAlister), 40 (Barros & Barros); Science Photo Library 16 (Dr E Walker), 18 (Damien Lovegrove), 25 bottom (A Glauberman), 29 (Jim Selby), 35 (Wesley Bocxe), 37 (Cordelia Molloy), 38 (BSIP Laurent), 39 (Tek Image), 41 (Cordelia Molloy), 43 (Will & Deni McIntyre); Stock Market *front cover* main image, 1, 5 (Robert Cerri), 9, 13, 19, 23, 26, 27 (Roy McMahon), 45; Tony Stone Images *cover band* middle (Andy Sacks), 6 (David Harry Stewart), 7 (Steve Taylor), 8 (Jean-Marc Truchet), 12 (Peter Dokus), 14 (Chad Slattery), 17 (Douet/TSI Imaging), 21 (Tim Hazael), 31 bottom (Simon Norfolk), 33 (Demetrio Carrasco), 34 (David Young Wolff), 36 (Zigy Kaluzny), 44 (Mark Harwood); The artwork on the cover and on pages 15 and 25 is by Michael Posen.

CONTENTS

WHAT IS A DRUG?

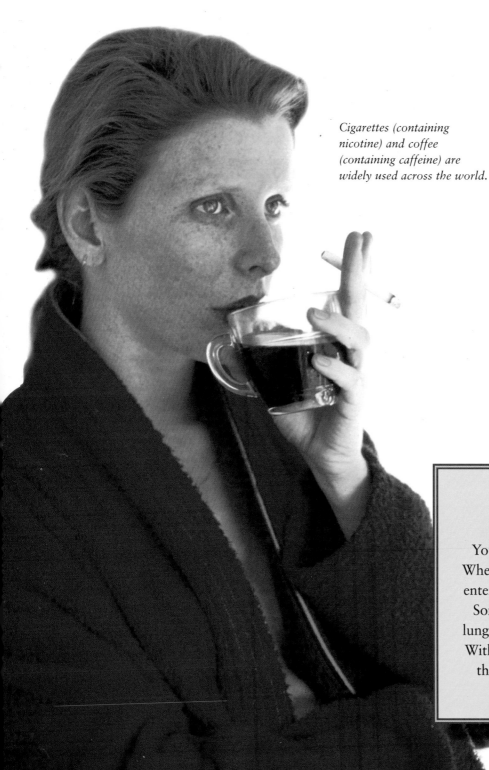

Cigarettes (containing nicotine) and coffee (containing caffeine) are widely used across the world.

A drug is a substance or chemical that affects the way your body or your mind works. Some drugs are artificially-made, others come from plants, minerals, even animals.

DRUGS IN HISTORY

Human beings have used drugs for thousands of years as medicines, to change the way they experience the world, or simply for pleasure. Over 10,000 years ago, American Indians used mescal beans as a stimulant. The Chinese have had herbal medicines for more than 5,000 years.

HOW PEOPLE TAKE DRUGS

You can take drugs in various ways. When you drink or swallow them, they enter the bloodstream via the stomach. Some are smoked or inhaled via the lungs, others administered by injection. With patches, suppositories or creams, the active ingredients are absorbed through the skin.

WHAT ARE DRUGS?

When someone mentions drugs, you probably think of illegal substances like heroin, cocaine or cannabis, but there are many other kinds of drugs. Chances are, you have taken several yourself. Most people have had aspirin or paracetamol for a headache, or antibiotics for an infection.
If you drink coffee, tea, coke or even eat chocolate, you will have consumed a stimulant drug called caffeine. Two of the most common drugs taken by adults are alcohol and tobacco.

Some drugs derive from things designed for other purposes. Solvents, for instance, used widely in glues and other household products, can have powerful effects when inhaled.

WHERE DO WE GET DRUGS?

New drugs are discovered every day. Medicines are often made up from chemicals in a laboratory, but many are extracted from plants. One reason people are so concerned about destruction of the Amazon rain forest is because so many of our drugs have come from plants discovered there.

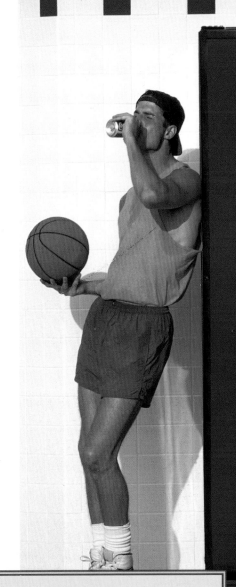

When it was first manufactured, Coca-Cola contained the drug cocaine, which is now illegal. Coke still contains the stimulant drug caffeine, which is quite legal and is also found in coffee and tea.

WHERE DRUGS COME FROM

Name	What is it?	Where does it come from?
Aspirin	Painkiller	Bark of the willow tree
Caffeine	Stimulant	Coffee beans, cocoa and tea leaves
Cannabis	Recreational drug	*Cannabis sativa* plant
Digitalis	Heart drug	Foxgloves
Taxol	Anti-cancer drug	Yew trees
Tobacco	Recreational drug	*Nicotiana tabacum* plants

LEGAL AND ILLEGAL DRUGS

Drugs are strong substances, which can have powerful effects on our bodies and our minds. For that reason, many countries and cultures have forbidden some drugs, either by religion or law. In most Western countries, drugs like heroin, cocaine, speed, ecstasy and cannabis are illegal to sell and to buy. In Muslim countries like Saudi Arabia, alcohol is illegal. Many illegal drugs have only been so for a relatively short time. Until earlier this century, cocaine was a main ingredient in Coca-Cola. In Britain opium, a relative of heroin, was freely available until the late eighteenth century. It was only when doctors became aware of their dangers and addictiveness that governments banned them.

Alcohol and cigarettes are widely regarded as 'social' drugs, meaning that groups of people can enjoy them together. People who become dependent on alcohol or cigarettes often find it hard to socialize without a drink or cigarette.

THE STRENGTH OF DRUGS

Whether a drug is legal or illegal doesn't necessarily relate to how powerful or dangerous it is. Too much alcohol or tobacco, for instance, can shorten your life considerably. Alcohol can also make you a danger to other people, especially if you drink and drive. Some people say this means we should legalize drugs like cannabis. They argue that it doesn't make sense to ban some, while other powerful and dangerous drugs are legal.

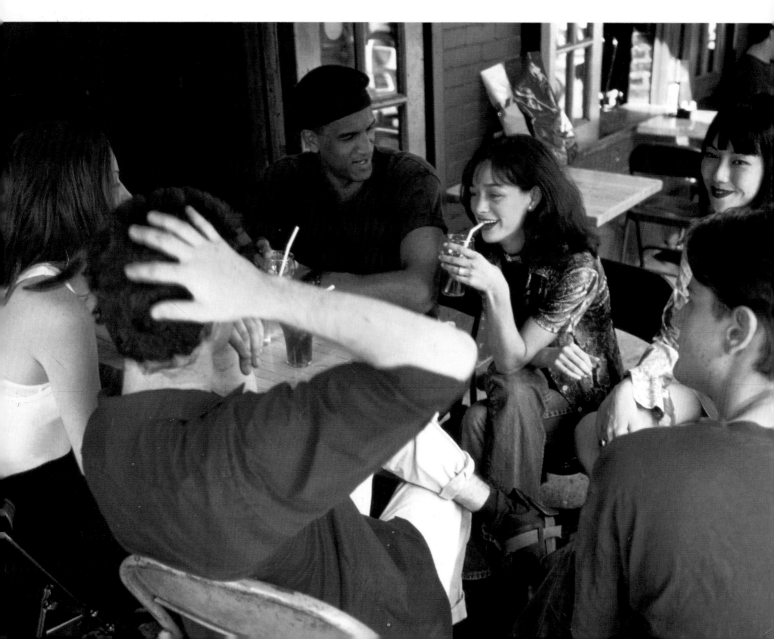

IS IT LEGAL?– UK AND US

DRUG	IS IT LEGAL?	CONSTRAINTS
Alcohol	Yes	Not available to children
Amphetamines (eg. speed)	Yes	As a prescribed appetite suppressant
Cannabis	No	Some US states allow possession of small amounts
Cocaine	No	
Ecstasy	No	
Hallucinogenic drugs (eg. LSD)	No	
Heroin	Yes	Only as a prescribed painkiller such as morphine
Sleeping tablets (eg. barbiturates)	Yes	Only on prescription
Tobacco	Yes	Not available to children
Tranquillizers (eg. Temazepam)	Yes	Only on prescription

CONTROL OF DRUGS

Medicinal drugs are controlled in different ways. Some, like painkillers, can be bought freely in shops and chemists. Most, however, are only available on prescription from a doctor.

The dried leaves and flowers of the cannabis plant, Cannabis sativa, have been smoked or chewed for their narcotic effect for centuries.

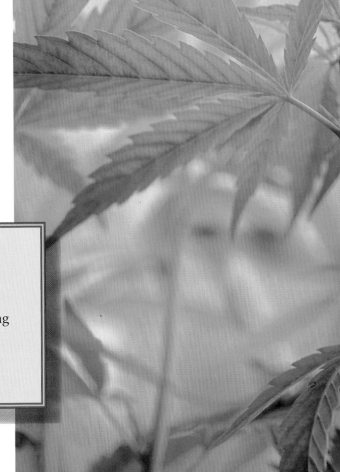

LEGALIZING CANNABIS

Cannabis is illegal in many countries, but pressure is increasing to legalize it for medicinal purposes. Smoking cannabis is said to bring great relief to sufferers of conditions like multiple sclerosis, arthritis and cancer.

ALCOHOL

WHAT IS ALCOHOL?

You can make alcohol from almost anything edible. Through a process called fermentation, sugars are converted into ethanol alcohol. This chemical is readily absorbed into the bloodstream and has a powerful effect on the body and mind. Stronger alcohols, called spirits, are made through distillation, where alcohol is heated to concentrate the ethanol.

Different societies use different ingredients and processes to make alcohol. In southern Europe, grapes are traditionally fermented to make wine – a process first introduced by the Romans. Northern European countries are famous for their beers brewed from grain and hops. Grapes are also the main ingredient of another famous French spirit called brandy. Other spirits include gin, vodka, and whisky.

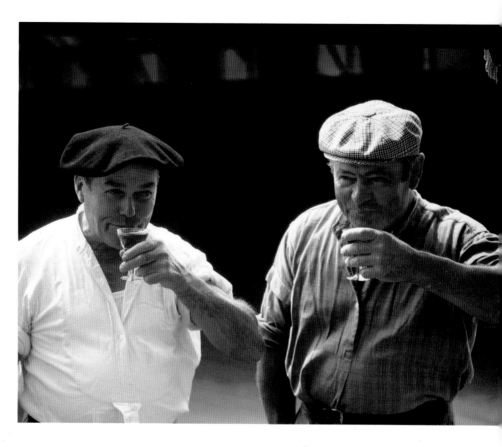

In countries such as Italy and France wine-making is a huge industry. People enjoy wine with their meals and when they are relaxing.

TYPES OF ALCOHOL

Today there are many different types of alcohol, all with varying strengths and tastes. Wine comes in many forms from fizzy champagnes to dark clarets. Beers can vary from pale German lagers to dark Irish stouts. By mixing different drinks, such as brandy and wine, you can produce other alcohols like sherry. Sometimes spirits are flavoured and sweetened to produce liqueurs like orange-flavoured Cointreau or aniseed-flavoured Pernod.

ALCOHOL STRENGTH

The strength of an alcoholic drink is known as its proof. Many producers put a percentage figure on the can or bottle which refers to the proof level, i.e. how much alcohol it contains. The higher the number, the less you can drink before the alcohol affects you.

ALCOPOPS

Recently brewers have started putting alcohol into traditional fizzy drinks. Known as 'alcopops', these come in lemonade, orangeade, cola, and many other flavours. They have been heavily criticized for deliberately appealing to younger people.

ATTITUDES TO ALCOHOL

Although alcohol is a drug, it doesn't generally have the bad reputation that other drugs have. Many countries see it as an important part of their culture; in France, for instance, enjoying fine wines has been a sign of education and good taste for hundreds of years. Other countries, however, have in the past tried to ban alcohol. In America the Prohibition banned alcohol for 13 years in the 1920s and 30s in an attempt to cut high drinking rates and resulting crime, poverty and violence.

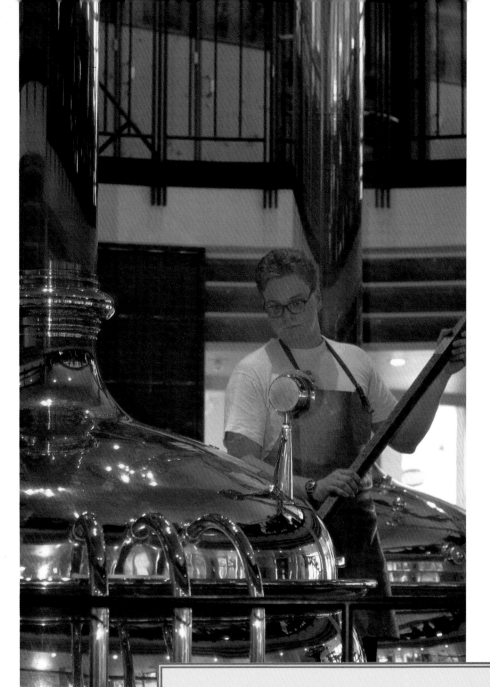

During the brewing process malt and other ingredients are mixed together, boiled and fermented.

HOW STRONG IS THAT DRINK?

Name	Type of Drink	Alcohol Content
Alcopop	Soft drink with alcohol added	4%–8%
Beer	Fermented mixture of grains and water	3%–10%
Liqueurs	Sweetened and flavoured spirits	20%–40%
Spirits	Alcoholic drink concentrated by distillation	38%–45%
Wine	Fermented grape juice	8%–14%

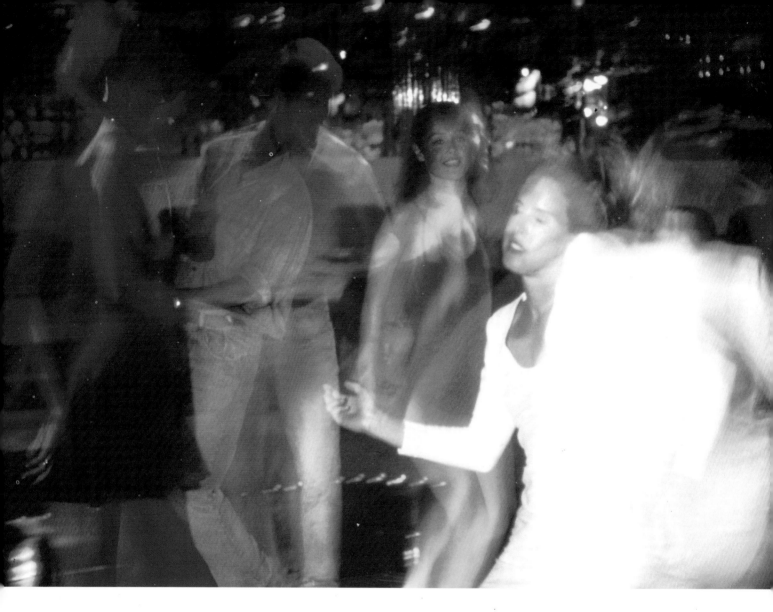

HOW DOES ALCOHOL AFFECT MY BODY?

Although it comes in different forms and strengths, alcohol has basically the same effects when you drink it. At first these may be pleasant. You may feel rather warm, light-headed and relaxed.

However, the more you drink, the worse you will feel. As more alcohol enters your bloodstream, you will find it increasingly difficult to perform physical tasks.

You will lose your coordination and sense of balance, knocking things over and feeling unsteady on your feet. Your speech will become slurred and difficult for other people to understand.

One of the most common symptoms of having drunk too much is the sensation that the room is spinning. This comes with a sick feeling in the stomach and usually means that the person is going to be physically sick.

ALCOHOL IN THE BLOOD

When alcohol enters your stomach, it is quickly absorbed into the blood. This travels quickly up to the brain, where it interferes with brain function. This is what leads to so many physical and mental symptoms.

THE EFFECTS OF ALCOHOL

Being very drunk is highly unpleasant, both for you and those around you. You will probably vomit, and may lose control of your bladder. Eventually you will collapse and fall asleep until your body has been able to process some of the alcohol.

DANGERS OF ALCOHOL

If you drink a lot very quickly, alcohol can kill. It can affect the brain so badly that the heart or breathing stops. You also run the risk of choking if you are sick. Every night, hospitals treat people who have drunk too much.

People who have drunk far too much can get alcohol poisoning. In cases like this hospitals have to pump the person's stomach to remove the alcohol.

BLOOD ALCOHOL LEVELS

The amount of alcohol you have drunk can be measured, as milligrams (mg) of alcohol per 100 millilitres (ml) of blood. The measurement is related to how you feel and react. The effects also depend on your sex, size, age, how much you have eaten and how used you are to drinking.

BLOOD ALCOHOL (mg/100ml)	EFFECT ON A MODERATE DRINKER
20	Usually feel relaxed and able to 'let go' slightly
60	Unable to make sensible decisions
100	Tend to be clumsy and unable to walk straight
180	Very drunk and unmanageable; may later not be able to remember what has happened
300	Often spontaneously incontinent. Possibly in coma.
500	Likely to die without medical help.

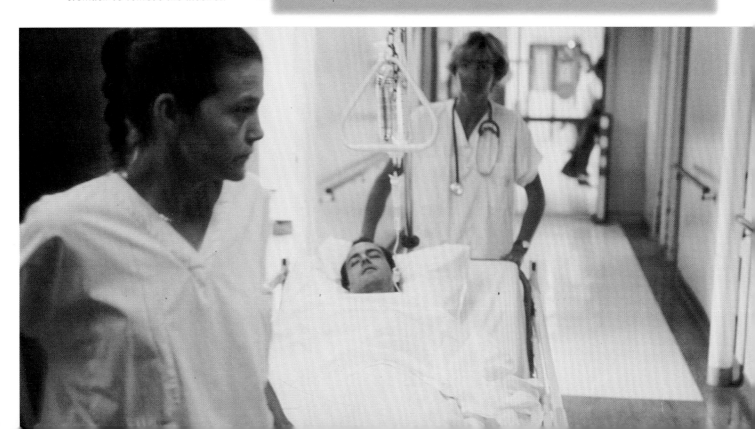

HOW ALCOHOL AFFECTS MY MIND

Alcohol also has powerful effects on the mind, altering your mood and the way you react. At first, you may feel more sociable, happy and confident. This is one reason people like to drink, especially when they're socialising.

People who drink too much regularly can become an embarrassment to their friends because of their unpredictable and drunken behaviour.

The more you drink, however, the worse you will feel. Alcohol is a depressant, and can make you feel more anxious or sad than normal. It affects your judgement, making you more likely to take risks. You can become paranoid and aggressive, misinterpreting what those around you say and do. Eventually you may be unable to recognize people, or even remember things like your own phone number. Alcohol can affect you so much that you may do things you would not normally consider.

This can have tragic consequences. Many crimes, murders, suicides and unwanted pregnancies occur when someone is drunk.

WHAT'S IN THAT DRINK?

You can judge how much you have drunk using units of alcohol. One unit of alcohol is the equivalent of one glass of wine, half a pint of average strength beer, or one measure of spirits.

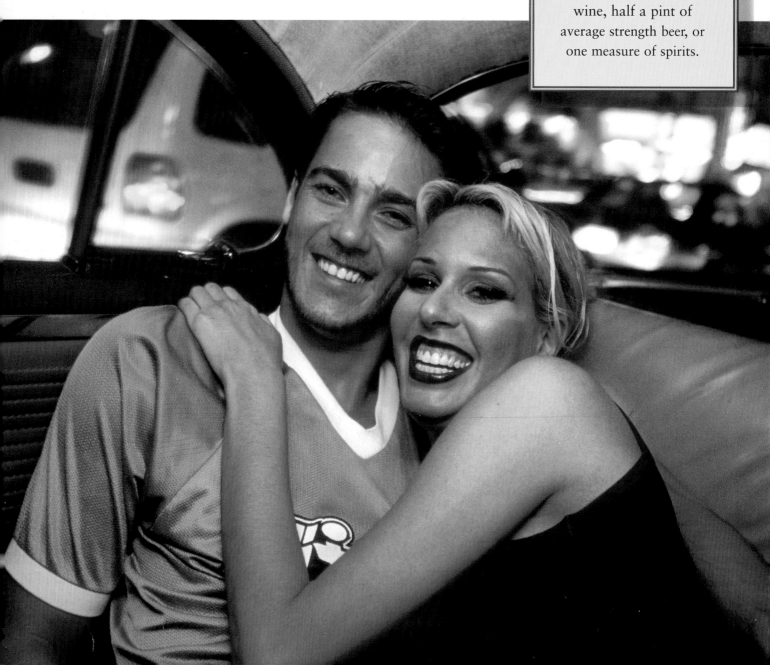

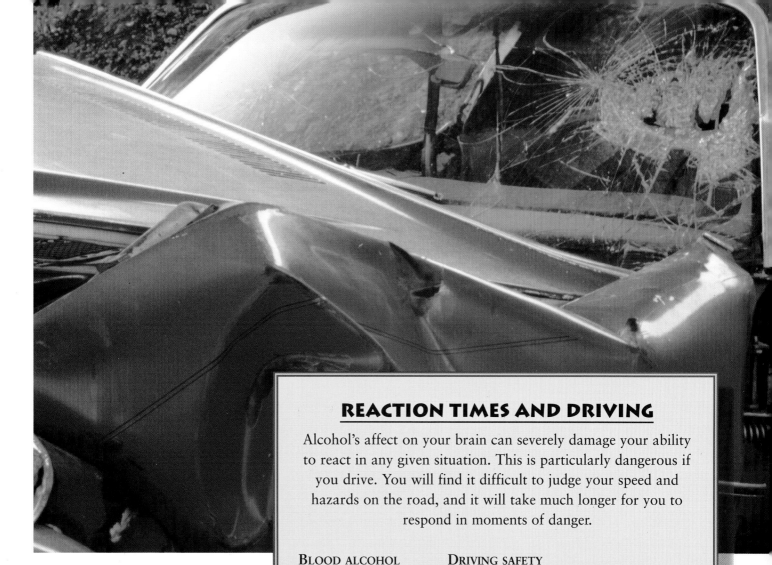

Despite advertising campaigns, every Christmas in the UK and US alcohol-related road accidents increase dramatically. People take risks driving when they are over the legal alcohol limit.

MEMORY LOSS

Most mental effects quickly reverse once the alcohol has left your body. However, your memory may be permanently damaged. People who get very drunk often wake up the next morning unable to remember what they did the night before.

REACTION TIMES AND DRIVING

Alcohol's affect on your brain can severely damage your ability to react in any given situation. This is particularly dangerous if you drive. You will find it difficult to judge your speed and hazards on the road, and it will take much longer for you to respond in moments of danger.

BLOOD ALCOHOL (mg/100ml)	DRIVING SAFETY
20–50	Tendency to take greater risks than normal and slight difficulty in judging speed.
50–79	It takes longer to react to danger so it may take longer to stop if necessary. Liable to drive too fast and misjudge distance.
80 and above	Your vision is impaired, you may not notice pedestrians, cars or other hazards. You are driving very badly by now.

The present UK legal limit for blood alcohol while driving is 80mg/100ml.

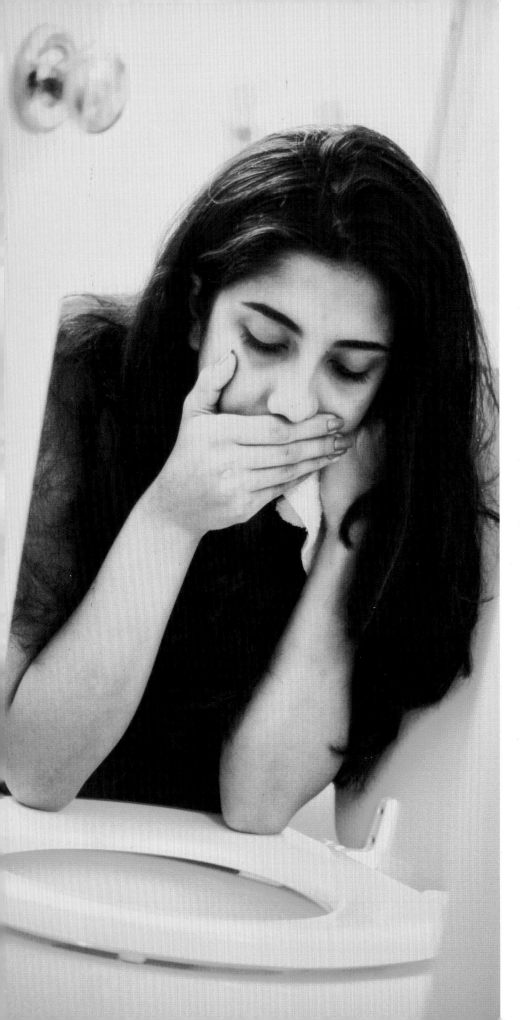

DRINKING TOO MUCH

You may have heard adults complain about hangovers. Although they may joke about it, drinking too much can make people feel very ill the next day, and it can take days for their bodies to recover.

WHAT IS A HANGOVER?

Various things cause hangovers. Alcohol moves water out of body cells, leading to dehydration, which causes headaches. It upsets the stomach, making people feel sick. It destroys vital vitamins and lowers blood sugar, which is why hangovers often make people feel hungry. Alcohol also strains the liver and stops you sleeping properly, which leaves you feeling exhausted and depressed. Generally a hangover feels like having been poisoned, which is exactly the case.

DOES EVERYONE SUFFER FROM HANGOVERS?

How bad someone feels depends mainly on how much they drink, although most people find hangovers get worse with age.

The liver is in the abdomen, below the diaphragm, and is attached to the stomach. It helps to digest and absorb fats and deals with the products of digestion. It also removes the poisons from substances like drugs and alcohol.

Blood from the intestines enters through the portal vein, and oxygenated blood from the heart enters via the hepatic artery. After being processed, blood leaves the liver through the hepatic vein, and waste products drain through the bile duct to the gall bladder.

ALCOHOL AND YOUR LIVER

The liver is the organ in your body which breaks down and eliminates poisons like alcohol. It has been likened to a car with one gear which just goes at one speed – the liver can only burn up one unit of alcohol an hour. Liver cells which have too much alcohol to process die and are replaced by fatty tissue.

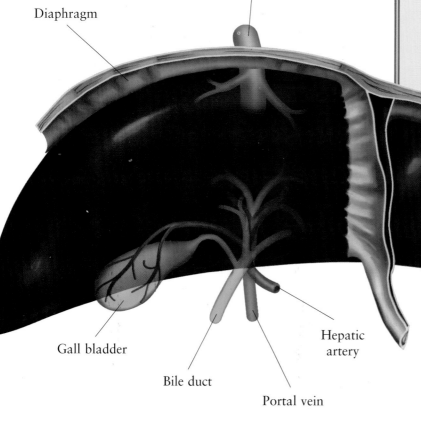

Hepatic vein

Diaphragm

Gall bladder

Bile duct

Hepatic artery

Portal vein

Many adults try to avoid a hangover by not mixing different types of drinks, eating well beforehand or while drinking, and drinking plenty of non-alcoholic fluids to counteract dehydration.

IS THERE A CURE?

There are many reputed cures for hangovers, but time, rest, plenty of fluids and healthy food is the best way to help the body recover. Painkillers like aspirin may also relieve headaches and antacids settle a queasy tummy. Of course, the best way to avoid a hangover is not to drink in the first place.

DID YOU KNOW?

Each year alcohol misuse leads to:
- ★ In the UK: 8–14 million lost working days.
  At least £50 million in related crime costs.
  Over £150 million a year in health expenditure.
- ★ In the US: $25 billion in related injuries and illness.
  Over 40% of work accidents.

LONG-TERM EFFECTS OF ALCOHOL

Although alcohol can make you feel bad the next day, drinking too much over a long period can make you very ill indeed. Drinking heavily over a number of years puts great strain on the liver, which can become so scarred that it no longer works properly. This is known as cirrhosis. Alcohol can also contribute to liver cancer.

ALCOHOL-RELATED DISEASES

Heavy drinking also contributes to other conditions like heart disease, hepatitis and stomach problems such as bleeding and ulcers. It can cause men to become sexually impotent (see glossary), and by interfering with the balance of hormones in the body increases the risk of breast cancer in women. Mothers who drink heavily when pregnant can severely damage their unborn child; in the US many babies are born with various deformities known as fetal alcohol syndrome.

This picture shows a cirrhosed liver. Cirrhosis is a disease – often caused by heavy alcohol consumption – in which scars break up the structure of the liver. The symptoms of cirrhosis of the liver are vomiting blood, mental confusion and jaundice.

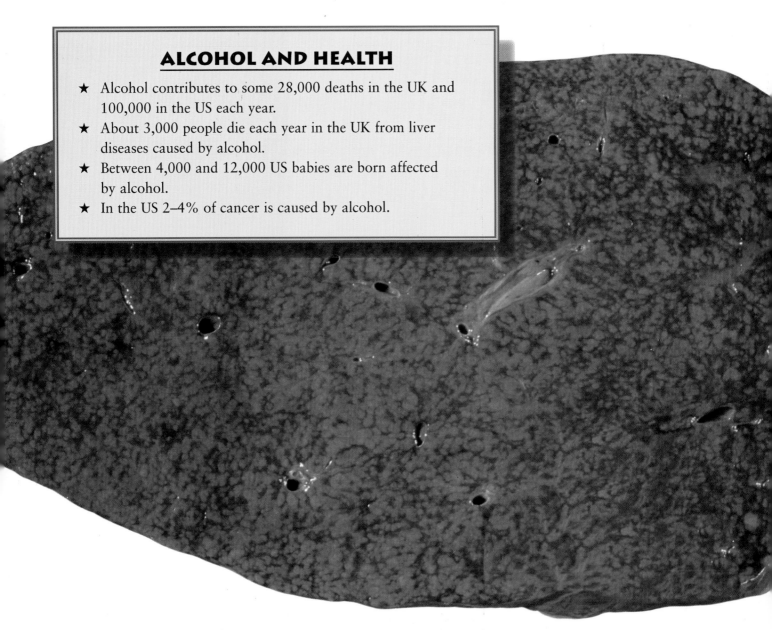

ALCOHOL AND HEALTH

★ Alcohol contributes to some 28,000 deaths in the UK and 100,000 in the US each year.
★ About 3,000 people die each year in the UK from liver diseases caused by alcohol.
★ Between 4,000 and 12,000 US babies are born affected by alcohol.
★ In the US 2–4% of cancer is caused by alcohol.

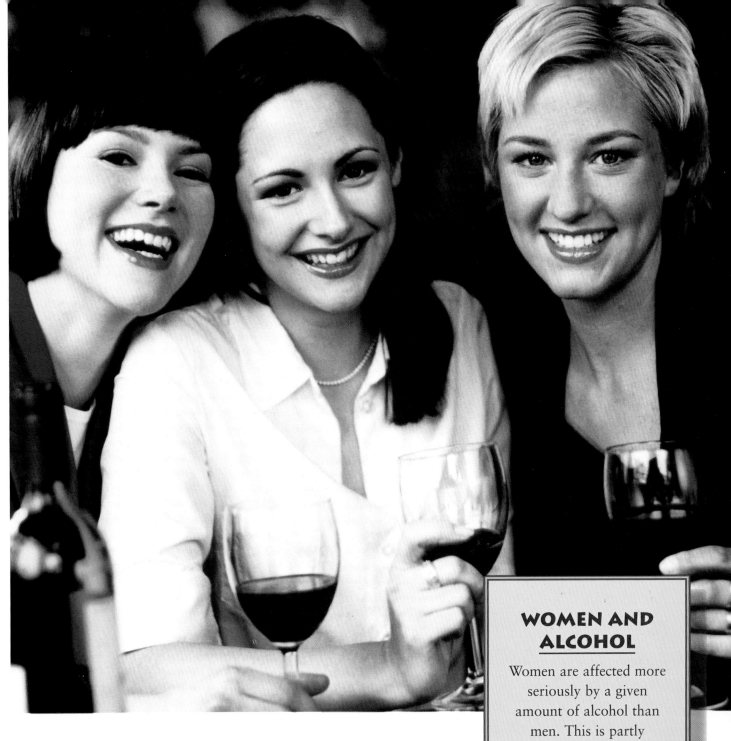

ALCOHOL AND WEIGHT-GAIN

Alcohol is also very fattening. It is loaded with calories which go straight into your bloodstream. A pint of beer, for instance, contains 180 calories, as much as an average chocolate bar. Heavy drinkers can develop malnutrition,

People often forget to include their alcohol intake when they are counting calories. Just a few glasses of wine or a couple of beers can be as calorific as an entire meal.

because they get all their energy from alcohol instead of food, and alcohol lacks essential vitamins and minerals.

WOMEN AND ALCOHOL

Women are affected more seriously by a given amount of alcohol than men. This is partly because they are smaller, which concentrates the alcohol in their blood. Women also store more fat than men – as alcohol can't dissolve in fat, it remains more active in their bodies.

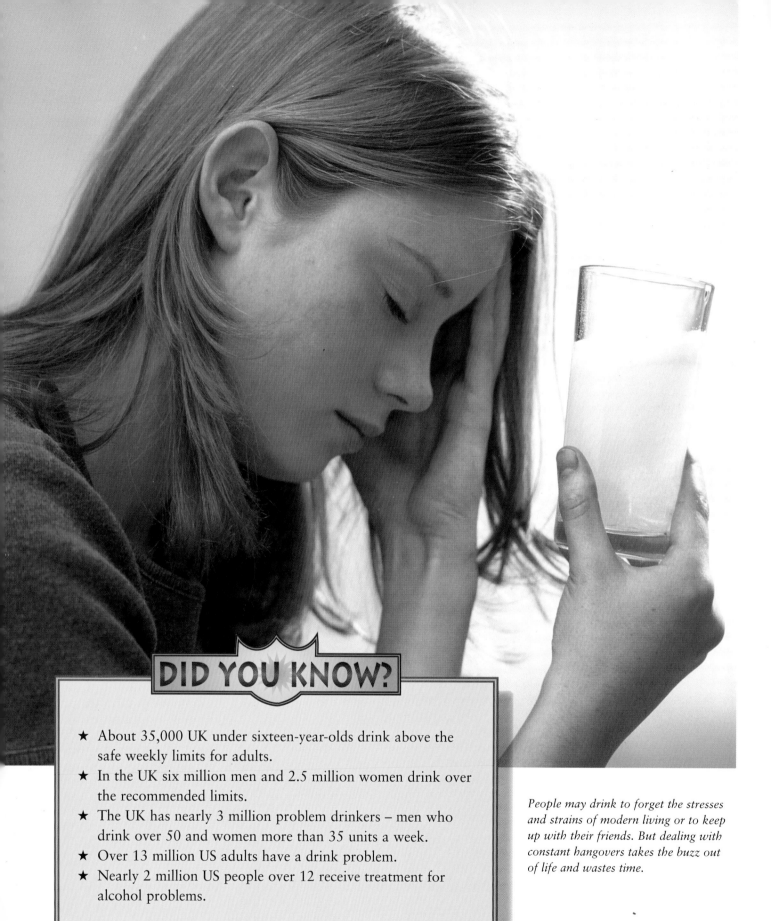

DID YOU KNOW?

★ About 35,000 UK under sixteen-year-olds drink above the safe weekly limits for adults.

★ In the UK six million men and 2.5 million women drink over the recommended limits.

★ The UK has nearly 3 million problem drinkers – men who drink over 50 and women more than 35 units a week.

★ Over 13 million US adults have a drink problem.

★ Nearly 2 million US people over 12 receive treatment for alcohol problems.

People may drink to forget the stresses and strains of modern living or to keep up with their friends. But dealing with constant hangovers takes the buzz out of life and wastes time.

WHAT IS ALCOHOLISM?

People who drink heavily for a long time can become addicted to alcohol. Those who develop an emotional or physical dependency on drink are known as alcoholics. No one is exactly sure why they become dependent. It could be a genetic tendency; alcoholism sometimes runs in families. It may be that heavy drinkers have psychological or other problems from which drink provides a temporary escape. Some experts, however, see alcoholism as a kind of disease.

ALCOHOL DEPENDENCY

Alcoholics, also known as problem or dependent drinkers, face more than just health problems. They may be unable to work properly, and can even lose their jobs. Drinking heavily inevitably affects their relationships with their families. Alcoholics may develop money problems or get into trouble with the police. They may then drink more heavily to get away from these problems.

Being an alcoholic can be very lonely. The desire for alcohol becomes overpowering and friendships and family are often neglected in favour of finding the next drink.

GIVING UP

Treatment programmes for alcohol addiction can be very effective. Some people go to 'drying out' clinics for help; others join groups like Alcoholics Anonymous for support in giving up. Alcoholics Anonymous has over two million members throughout the world.

SIGNS OF ALCOHOLISM

Alcoholism usually takes years to develop. Early signs include constantly needing to have drink available, and being unusually resistant to its effects. In the later stages, however, people gradually lose control over their drinking. They may need to have a drink as soon as they get up in the morning.

Once they start drinking they may well carry on until they are very drunk, known as binge drinking. Alcoholics often suffer from unpleasant conditions like shaking, various body pains and redness in the face. They can experience severe withdrawal effects if they suddenly stop. Unlike coming off other drugs, sudden alcohol withdrawal can actually kill.

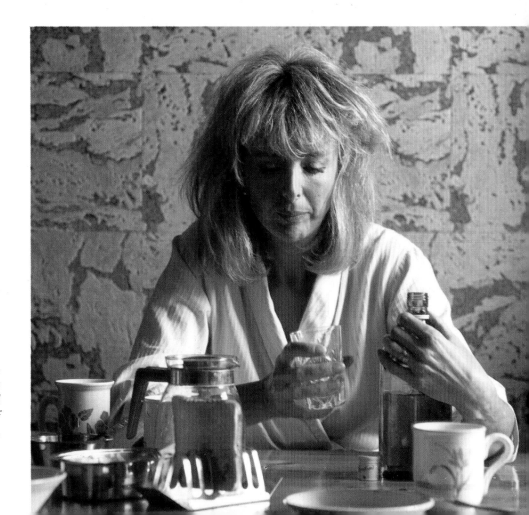

SMOKING

WHAT IS IN A CIGARETTE?

Cigarettes are made mainly from tobacco, the dried leaf the plant *Nicotiana tabacum*. Tobacco originated in Central America. There is evidence of smoking in the Mayan civilization there as long ago as AD 500. More than 600 substances are approved as cigarette additives in the UK. Many of them are secret ingredients designed to give each brand a distinctive flavour.

Today tobacco-growing is one of the largest industries in the world.

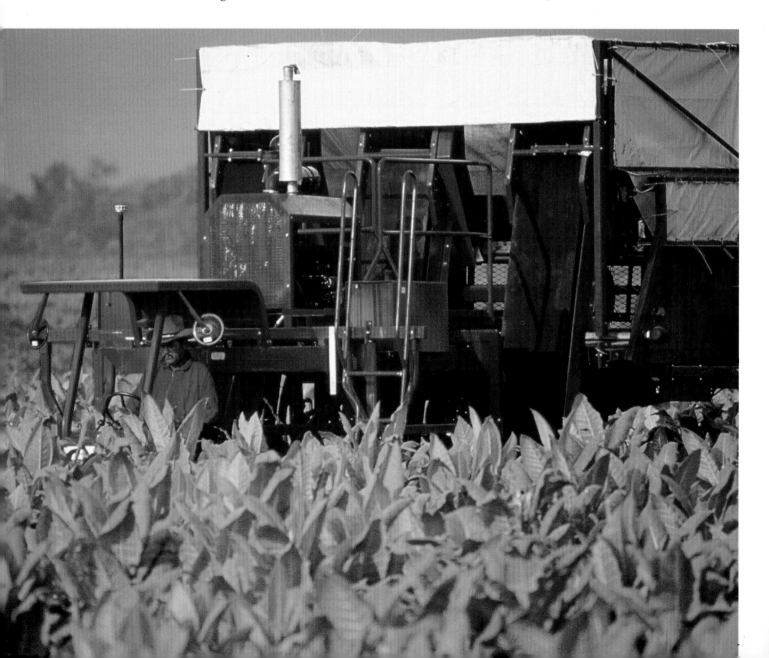

Recently tobacco companies have been accused of deliberately adding flavours like cocoa, vanilla and liquorice to cigarettes to attract young smokers. There is no obligation for cigarette manufacturers to describe these additives on the packet.

CHEMICALS IN TOBACCO

The main components of cigarettes include nicotine, a powerful drug which quickly leads to addiction. Carbon monoxide, the same gas that comes out of car exhausts, is the principal gas in cigarette smoke. Other chemicals include many that have links with cancer in humans, such as arsenic, benzene, cadmium, and formaldehyde.

THE COST OF CIGARETTES

Cigarettes are expensive, particularly in the UK, where government taxation on tobacco is high. With 20 King-size cigarettes costing around £3.30 in 1999, smoking a packet a day over 20 years will cost some £25,000 – assuming that prices don't rise further. That would buy a small house in many areas, or a top-of-the-range car.

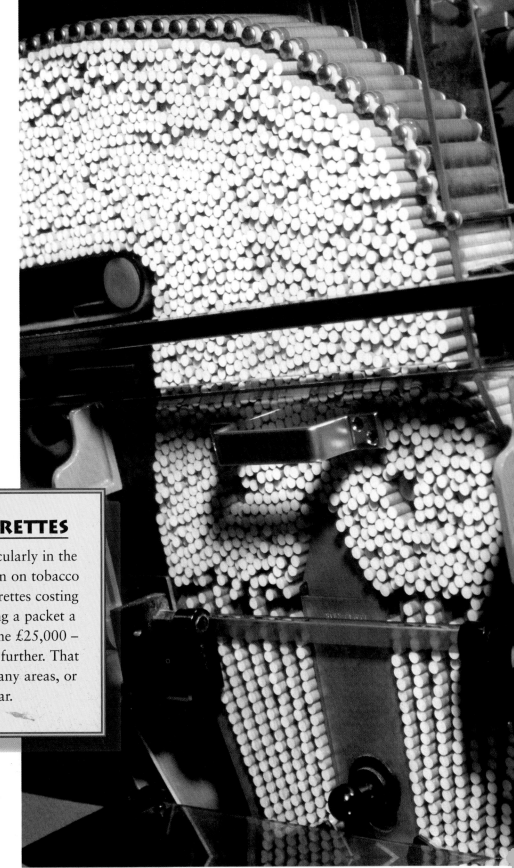

The packing machine at the end of the manufacturing line fills countless packets with cigarettes for the world market.

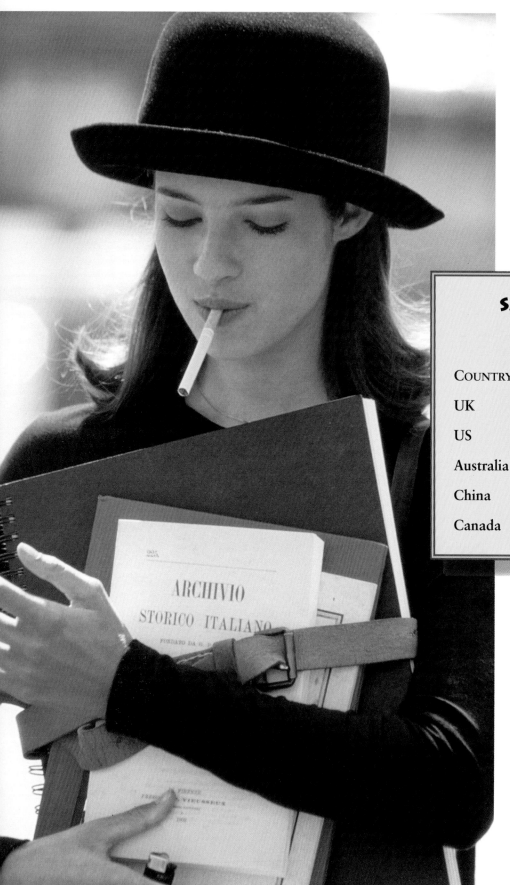

WHAT HAPPENS WHEN I SMOKE?

When you take a puff on a cigarette, many things happen. In just a few seconds, nicotine is delivered to the brain. This stimulates the body's central nervous system, increasing the heart rate and blood pressure. Smoking also reduces the appetite and lowers skin temperature.

SMOKING RATES WORLDWIDE

COUNTRY	NUMBERS OF SMOKERS
UK	12,000,000
US	50,000,000
Australia	3,500,000
China	300,000,000
Canada	6,000,000

CARBON MONOXIDE

Carbon monoxide gas, found in high concentrations in cigarette smoke, combines readily with haemoglobin, the substance in the blood that carries oxygen around the body.

Most smokers say that at certain times of the day, such as after a meal, they always crave a cigarette. Breaking these habits is the key to quitting smoking.

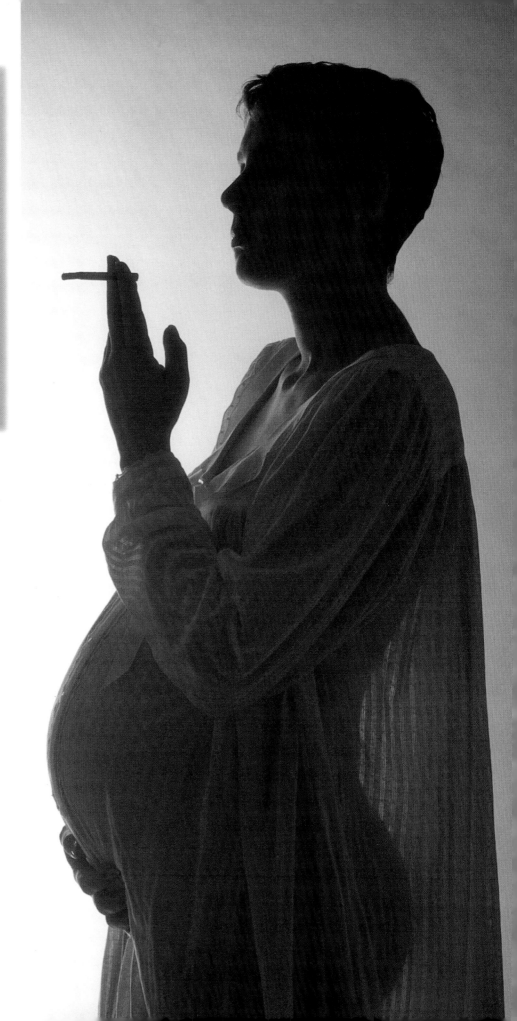

PREGNANCY AND TOBACCO

Pregnant women who smoke are putting their baby's health at serious risk. The baby is more likely to be born prematurely, or to die in the womb or shortly after birth. Babies born to smokers are often smaller. They get less oxygen in the womb, which makes their hearts beat faster and slows their growth.

In heavy smokers, up to 15 per cent of their blood can carry carbon monoxide instead of oxygen, depriving tissues and body cells from the oxygen they need to function. Long term shortage of oxygen can cause problems with the growth, repair and exchange of essential nutrients, increasing the risk of diseases like cancer.

If you are not used to smoking, you may notice other effects. Just one cigarette can make you feel sick, dizzy and may even make you vomit. These effects tend to wear off if you start smoking regularly.

Smoking – especially for pregnant women – is becoming less and less acceptable in the community. Laws have been passed in some of the states in the United States to prevent any smoking in public places.

WHY IS SMOKING SO BAD FOR MY HEALTH?

Everyone knows that smoking is bad for them, but not necessarily why. Smoking attacks your health in many ways. Carbon monoxide affects the electrical activity of the heart, encouraging fatty deposits to form on the artery walls. This increases the risk of heart attacks and other heart problems.

Smoking also raises the heart rate and blood pressure, which also increases the risk of heart attacks and bleeding in the brain, called strokes.

These are just some of the diseases that are more common in smokers than in non-smokers.

Strokes
Blood loss to the brain. Often fatal or severely disabling.

Tobacco amblyopia
Defective vision.

Chronic bronchitis
Inflammation of the bronchial tubes leading into the lungs, resulting in coughing, wheeziness and fever.

Mouth and throat cancer

Lung cancer

Aortic aneurysm
A swelling of the main artery in the body, with the risk of rupture and fatal blood loss.

Emphysema
An often fatal lung disease which destroys the walls of the air sacs.

Heart attack

Peptic ulcers
Raw and painful areas in the intestines.

Cancer of the cervix
(in women)

Lowered fertility

Gangrene
Death and decay of part of the body due to loss of blood supply when fatty deposits, caused by smoking, clog up the arteries.

Peripheral vascular disease
Disease of the arteries in the leg.

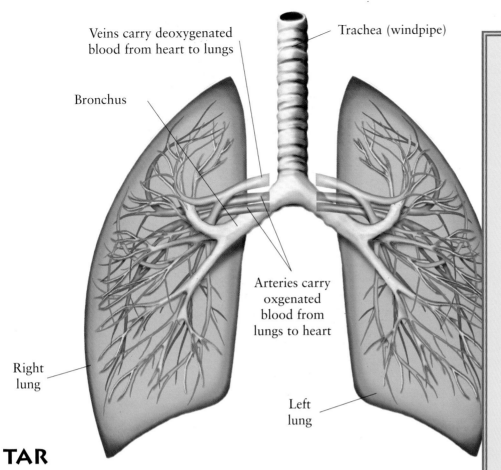

Veins carry deoxygenated blood from heart to lungs

Trachea (windpipe)

Bronchus

Arteries carry oxgenated blood from lungs to heart

Right lung

Left lung

TAR

Tar, one of the main by-products of smoking even in low-tar brands, is also a killer. About 70 per cent of the tar in inhaled cigarette smoke is deposited in the lungs, clogging them up and leading to coughs and breathlessness. Irritants in the tar also damage the delicate tissues of the lungs, increasing the risk of infection. Many of the chemicals present in tar are known to cause cancer, particularly lung cancer.

Above The lungs put oxygen into the blood and remove toxic carbon dioxide from it. Smoking leaves tar deposits on the lungs, damaging them and making them less effective.

This is a smoker's lung. It is darker and rougher than a non-smoker's lung and mis-shapen. Smoking inflames the lungs and scars them. It can also cause lung cancer.

PASSIVE SMOKING

For most people, breathing in other people's cigarette smoke causes 'minor' symptoms like watering eyes, itching nose and throat, and dizziness. But for some the effects are more serious. Babies and young children may suffer from more infections and serious chest conditions like bronchitis and pneumonia. People exposed to passive smoking over long periods are also at a 10–30 per cent increased risk of death from lung cancer.

DEATH RATES

Each year 120,000 people in the UK, and 500,000 in the US die from smoking-related disease. Even when smoking doesn't lead to serious illness, it causes everyday complaints like coughing, bad breath and shortness of breath.

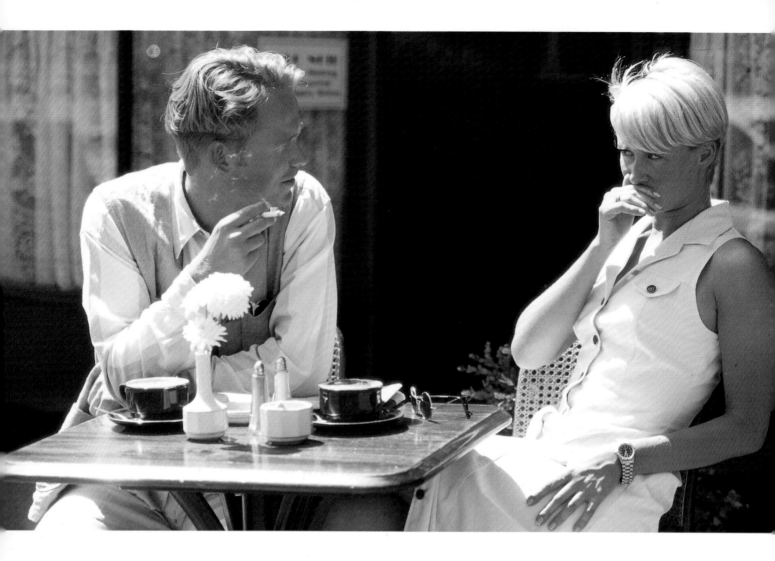

WHY DO PEOPLE BECOME ADDICTED?

Smoking is very addictive. You have a 90 per cent chance of getting hooked from smoking just a few cigarettes. This is mainly due to nicotine, which quickly produces effects on the brain when smokers are deprived of it. Smokers say that cigarettes make them feel more relaxed when they are tense, or more able to concentrate when they are tired, but much of this tenseness or tiredness is actually due to nicotine withdrawal.

SOCIAL PRESSURES TO SMOKE

This cycle of smoking and withdrawal can lead to chain-smoking, with heavy smokers getting through 40–60 cigarettes a day. But nicotine is not the only culprit. Young people often feel pressurised into smoking by friends or acquaintances. You may start off smoking just to feel included, but quickly end up addicted. Cigarette advertising, banned in many countries, also encourages people to associate smoking with being cool or successful.

Many people find the smoke from other people's cigarettes irritating and unpleasant.

Smokers often say they find smoking comforting, especially in times of stress or upset. Many people enjoy the ritual of lighting up over a coffee or after a meal. This is what we call psychological addiction. Giving up these habits can be as difficult as coping with the physical cravings.

MYTHS ABOUT SMOKING

Many people, girls in particular, start smoking to keep their weight down. Recent research, however, suggests that smoking in the longer term actually makes you fatter.

STARTING YOUNG

The first cigarettes smoked can feel and taste very unpleasant, yet many people start smoking in their teens. This is often because they feel that it makes them look older or 'cool'. Often people start simply because all their friends do. If someone comes from a smoking family, they may feel it is a natural part of growing up.

DID YOU KNOW?

★ In the UK, 450 children under 16 start smoking each day – each year 11–15-year-olds smoke over 1 billion cigarettes – almost a quarter of 15-year-olds are regular smokers.

★ In the US, more than 3000 under-18-year-olds take up smoking each day – at least four-and-a-half million under-18s smoke.

People may choose to smoke because they believe it makes them look grown-up or sophisticated. Very often these people become addicted to tobacco and then are unable to quit smoking when they want to.

WHAT HAPPENS WHEN YOU TRY TO GIVE UP?

All smokers know they would be better off if they gave up. Unfortunately, kicking the habit is not easy. Nicotine is as addictive as heroin, and it takes a lot of will-power to overcome the physical and psychological cravings. On average, seven out of ten smokers try and fail to quit at least twice. Sometimes people give up for years, only to light up again in a stressful situation.

WITHDRAWAL SYMPTOMS

That said, some 11 million UK and 40 million US smokers have given up. Most find that the first few days are the hardest, as nicotine withdrawal causes unpleasant symptoms such as lack of concentration, light-headedness, anxiety, coughing, hunger and strong cravings. These usually pass within a week or so.

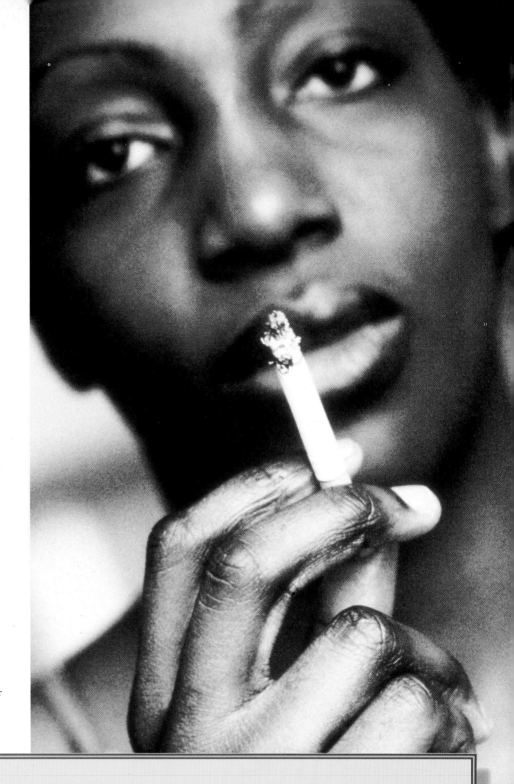

Most smokers would like to give up smoking, but the stresses and strains of life make it hard for them to do so.

A HELPING HAND

There are many products and services available to help you give up. These range from nicotine patches, gum and lozenges, which lessen the physical craving by giving the body small amounts of the drug, to psychological aids, such as hypnotism, to reduce the urge to smoke.

AFTER THE LAST PUFF

TIME	EFFECTS ON THE BODY
20 minutes later	Blood pressure and pulse return to normal
One day later	Lungs start to clear out mucus and other deposits
Two days later	Body is clear of nicotine
Three days later	Breathing becomes easier
2–12 weeks later	Circulation improves
3–9 months later	Lungs become more efficient
1 year later	Excess risk of heart disease is halved
10 years later	Risk of lung cancer reduced by half
15 years later	Risk of death from lung cancer, heart disease and stroke return to non-smoking levels.

QUITTING

But breaking the psychological dependency on smoking is just as difficult. People often have to change their routines and avoid places they associate with smoking. Being with other smokers is particularly hard when you are trying to quit. Within several months, however, most people find that even the urge to smoke disappears. Many even start to find smoking unpleasant.

Nicotine patches are just one of the many different methods of quitting that are on offer to smokers.

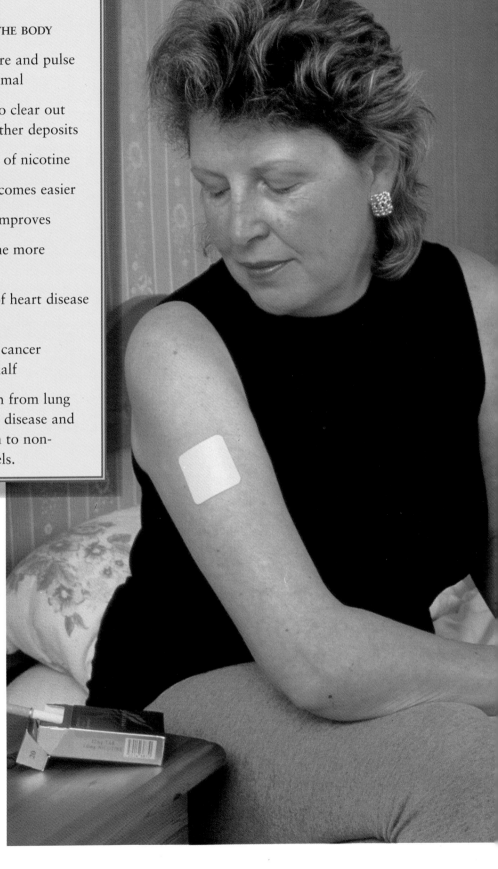

ILLEGAL DRUGS

WHAT HAPPENS WHEN YOU TAKE AN ILLEGAL DRUG?

People take illegal drugs for many reasons – because their friends do, for fun, to escape their problems, or simply out of curiosity. But most people have no idea what these drugs do to their bodies or minds. Drugs act in different ways. Stimulants, such as cocaine, ecstasy and speed, act on your body's central nervous system and increase brain activity. Depressants, like alcohol, solvents, and sedatives, also affect the central nervous system, but actually slow down brain activity.

Hallucinogens like cannabis, LSD and magic mushrooms, influence the mind, distorting the way you see and hear things. Exactly how a drug affects you depends on many things – like your size, whether you have taken anything else, such as alcohol, and how used you are to that particular drug. It also depends on how you take it.

TYPES OF ILLEGAL DRUGS

Drug	Street names	Usual form	How taken
Amphetamine	Speed, whizz, uppers	Powder or tablets	Swallowed, sniffed, injected, smoked
Cannabis	Blow, dope, ganja, puff, weed	Brown/black resin or grass	Smoked or eaten
Cocaine	Charlie, snow, crack	White powder, crystals	Sniffed or smoked
Ecstasy	E, XTC, doves	Pills	Swallowed
Heroin	Smack, horse, skag junk, gear	Brown or white powder	Injected, sniffed or smoked
LSD	Acid, trips	Tablets, impregnated paper	Swallowed
Magic mushrooms	Shrooms, mushies	Dried/fresh mushrooms	Eaten
Sedatives	Barbiturates, Temazepam	Tablets	Swallowed
Solvents		Glue, lighter fuel, nail varnish, petrol, aerosols	Inhaled

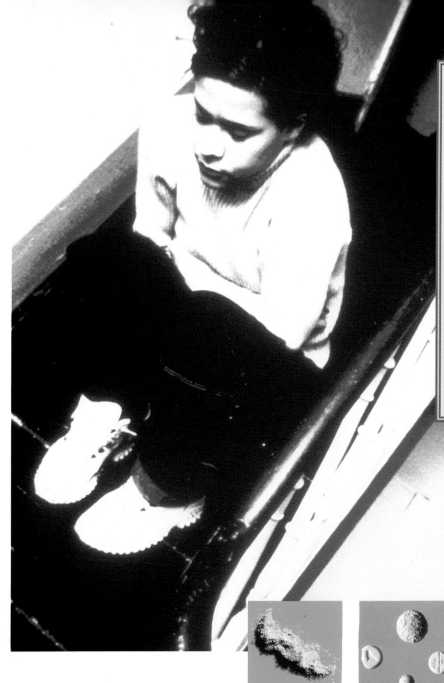

It is impossible to tell whether the drug you are buying has been properly manufactured or not. A bad reaction can produce frightening symptoms in people.

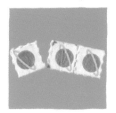
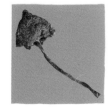
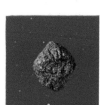
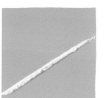
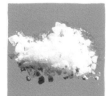
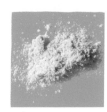

Injecting or snorting a drug tends to have a faster and more powerful effect than swallowing one.

KNOWING WHAT YOU'RE GETTING

Another problem with illegal drugs is that you can never be sure exactly what is in them. Many cases of overdose or harm occur because a drug is too pure, or is contaminated with other substances.

From left to right, pictured are nine illegal drugs: heroin, esctasy, cannabis (grass), magic mushroom, LSD, cannabis resin, cocaine, crack and speed.

HOW CAN DRUGS MAKE YOU FEEL?

Many people drink alcohol because they like the taste, but most people take illegal drugs to make them feel different. These feelings depend on the drug. While ecstasy produces feelings of friendliness and happiness, cannabis can makes things seem funnier than usual and heightens enjoyment of food and music.

BAD REACTIONS

However, most illegal drugs can make you feel very bad indeed. You never know how you will react to an illegal or abused substance. You may feel fine, for instance, the first dozen times you take cannabis, then suddenly experience strong feelings of fear or paranoia. LSD and mushrooms in particular can produce 'bad trips' – extreme feelings of anxiety, fear, paranoia, even nightmare visions.

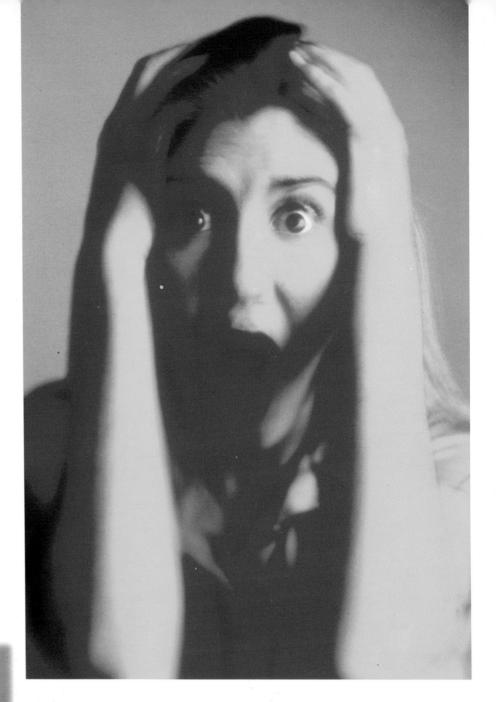

WHO TAKES DRUGS?

In the UK, drug use is highest in people from their mid-teens to their late twenties. In the population overall, about a third of people have taken drugs at some point in their life. For those aged 16–29, as many as 25 per cent have taken drugs within the last year.

Unfortunately, if you do have a bad reaction, all you can do is wait for the effects to wear off.

MOOD

A lot depends on the mood you are in when you take a drug. Cannabis heightens whatever you are feeling at the time, so if you are more anxious or depressed than usual, the drug can make you feel worse. As with alcohol, drugs

Above Paranoia is a common reaction to certain drugs. The person becomes afraid and thinks that they are being persecuted or chased.

Right In many nightclubs, owners are trying to prevent the trend in people taking ecstasy.

also affect your reactions. You will find it more difficult to control how you feel and what you do if something happens to you.

DRUGS AND THEIR EFFECTS

Drug	Good feelings	Bad feelings	How long it lasts
Amphetamines	Wakefulness, happiness	Anxiety, panic	3–4 hours
Cannabis	Relaxation, relieves boredom, enhances sensory awareness	Paranoia, panic	1–12 hours
Cocaine	Exhilaration, well-being, indifference to pain or tiredness	Insomnia	20–30 minutes Crack lasts 10–12 minutes
Ecstasy	Happiness, friendliness, energy, calmness	Nausea, fatigue and depression after use	Several hours
Heroin	Happiness, content, warmth, peacefulness	Nausea, vomiting	3–4 hours, depending on how taken
LSD/ mushrooms	Fascinating sound and visual hallucinations, euphoria	Waking nightmares, paranoia	12 hours
Sedatives	Calmness, relaxation	Nausea, vomiting	Several hours
Solvents	Hallucinations, euphoria	Hangovers, drowsiness	Few minutes

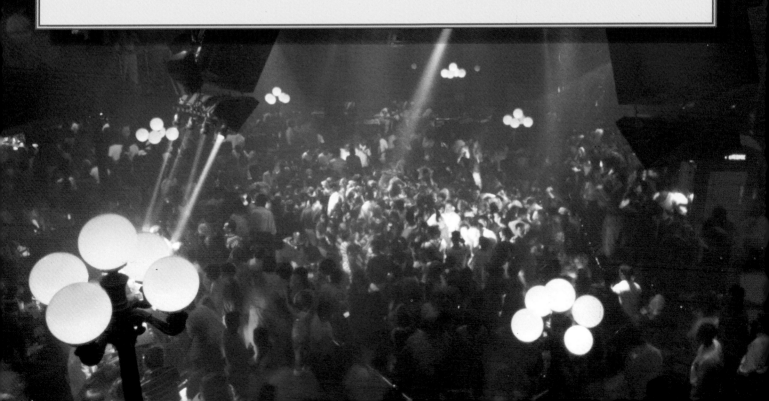

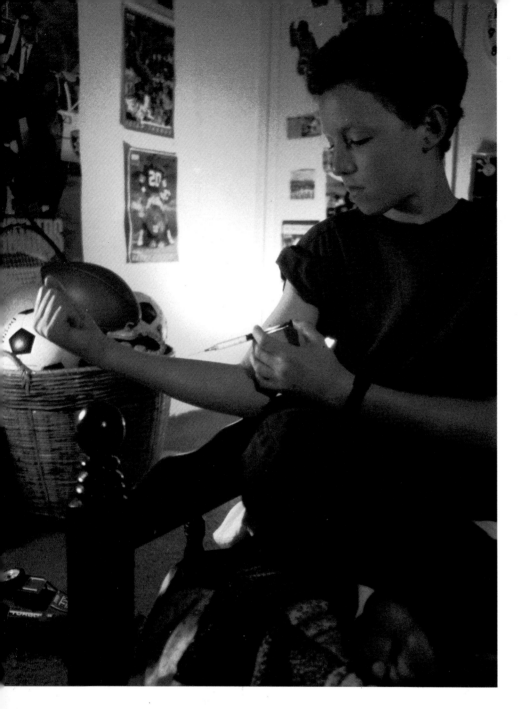

This boy is using a syringe to inject himself with drugs. Because there are very few physical symptoms, parents may not find out that their child is using drugs until he or she has become addicted.

METHADONE

Most Western countries have programmes to help people come off heroin and other drug addictions. Methadone can help some people addicted to heroin to come off the drug without feeling all the withdrawal symptoms. There are also residential centres where addicts can try to give up within a safe and supportive environment, or alternatives such as counselling, self-help groups, and educational activities.

WHY ARE SOME DRUGS ADDICTIVE?

Most illegal or abused substances are not addictive. If you take cannabis, ecstasy, amphetamines, LSD or solvents, for example, you can't become addicted to them in the same way you might to cigarettes or even alcohol, because your body won't come to depend on them.

PHYSICAL DEPENDENCY

Unfortunately, this is not true of heroin, cocaine, crack or sedatives. You can become physically dependent on these drugs, which means that you need them to feel well or normal, and you experience withdrawal symptoms if you suddenly stop taking them.

EXPERIMENTING WITH DRUGS

How quickly you become addicted depends on how much and how often you take them, as well as your personality and circumstances.

Many people do, for instance, experiment with heroin without becoming addicted; it may take several weeks or months of heavy use to become dependent. Crack cocaine, however is rapidly addictive.

However, just because you are not physically addicted to a drug, doesn't mean you're not dependent on it in other ways. If you feel you cannot enjoy yourself without smoking cannabis or taking ecstasy, then you have become psychologically dependent on the drug to function normally.

These vials contain white crack crystals. Crack comes from cocaine and is highly addictive and very strong. Crack users heat the crystals to produce a vapour which they then inhale.

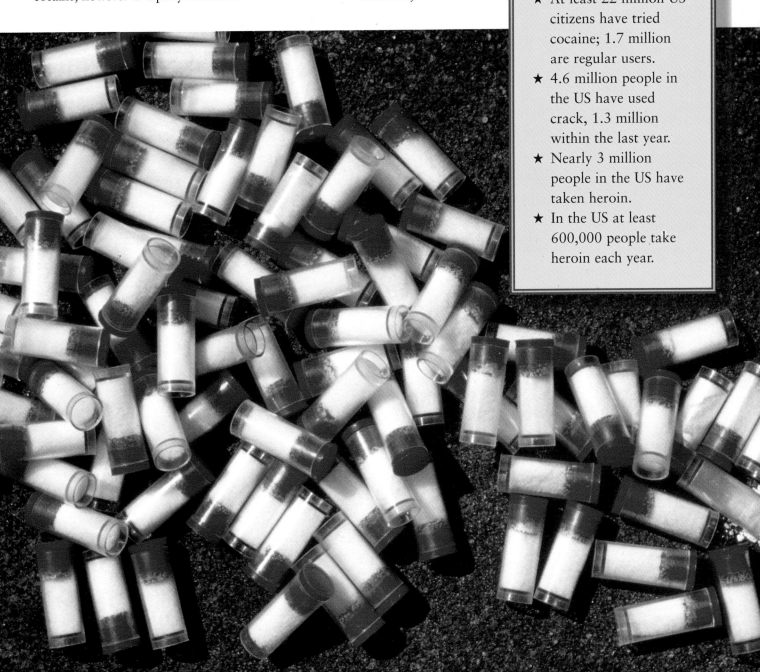

HEROIN/CRACK ADDICTION

★ In 1996, there were 43,372 registered UK heroin addicts – around 20–30 per cent of the total number of addicts.

★ Less than one per cent of the UK population use heroin and two per cent cocaine.

★ At least 22 million US citizens have tried cocaine; 1.7 million are regular users.

★ 4.6 million people in the US have used crack, 1.3 million within the last year.

★ Nearly 3 million people in the US have taken heroin.

★ In the US at least 600,000 people take heroin each year.

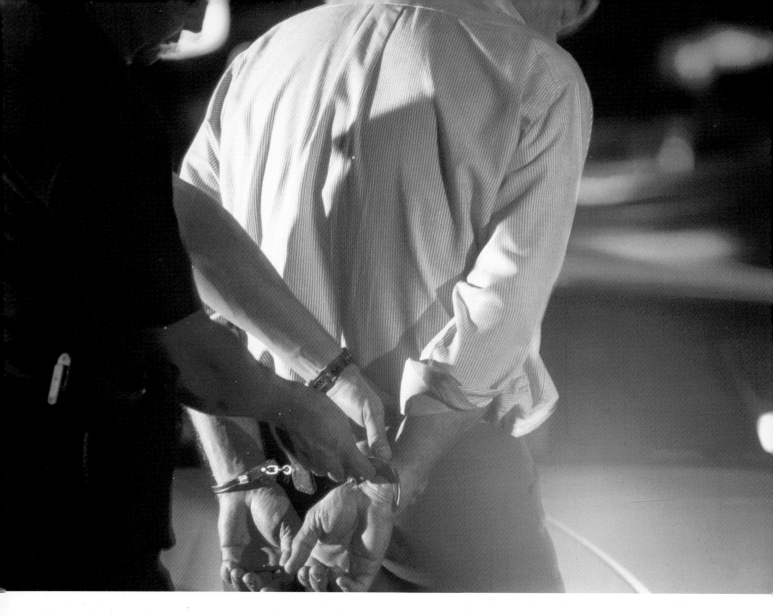

HOW CAN DRUGS AFFECT ME IN THE LONGER TERM?

Even if most drugs don't lead to addiction, they can be habit forming. The temptation is to take them more and more frequently. You may have heard the term 'there's no such thing as a free lunch'. This is particularly true of drugs. While no one would deny that taking them can make you feel good in the short term, over time they will take their toll on both your body and your mind.

Once a person becomes addicted to a drug, they will do anything to get their next fix – even break the law.

DRUGS AND CRIME

★ Long term drug use is extremely expensive. A lot of crime is committed to pay for drugs like heroin and crack.

★ Heroin and cocaine addicts need between £10,000 and £40,000 a year to pay for drugs.

★ The cost to victims of drug-related crime is over £2.5 billion per year.

★ In one area, over three months in 1997, 700 heroin addicts committed 70,000 criminal offences.

COMING DOWN

Some drugs like cocaine and ecstasy make you pay for the pleasure they give by leaving you feeling tired and depressed for several days afterwards. Over long term use, the physical effects of drugs can be greater.

Cocaine can cause heart problems, chest pain and even convulsions, and can permanently damage the lining of your nose. Ecstasy has been linked to liver and kidney problems. Long term use of amphetamines can put a strain on your heart. As with tobacco, smoking a lot of cannabis puts you at risk of throat and lung cancer.

PAYING THE PRICE

With many other drugs, however, the effects are more subtle. Smoking cannabis long term, for instance, often leads to a lack of motivation and feelings of apathy. It can also impair the ability to learn and concentrate, making it even harder to get on with life. One of the problems with illegal drugs is that they are not tested for safety in the same way as medical drugs. No one knows, therefore, what the long term effects of a drug may be, particularly for newer substances like ecstacy.

A razor blade is used to chop up speed (an amphetamine) into a fine powder which is then snorted.

DRUGS AND YOUR MENTAL HEALTH

Some drugs can permanently affect your mental health. LSD and magic mushrooms can lead to flashbacks, where you temporarily relive some aspect of your 'trip', even years afterwards. More worryingly, these hallucinogens can trigger severe mental health problems like depression and schizophrenia in vulnerable people. There is increasing evidence that ecstasy can permanently change the chemicals in your brain, making you more vulnerable to depression and anxiety.

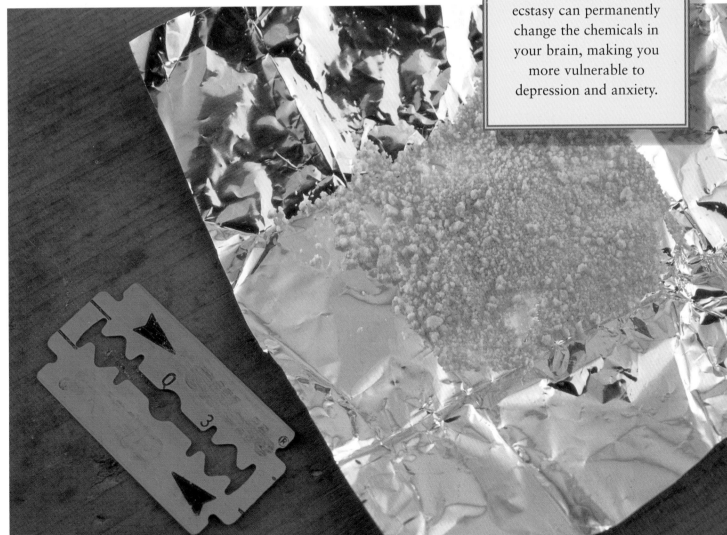

CAN DRUGS REALLY KILL ME?

People used to think that all drugs were extremely dangerous and taking them inevitably lead to addiction and death. Although this put a lot of people off drugs, many others discovered that this simply wasn't true.

Although many people use drugs recreationally without serious side-effects, for some it can end in tragedy.

DRUG DEATHS

The following table shows deaths caused by drugs in 1985–94 (not including drug related road deaths).

DRUG	DEATHS
Cocaine	67
Amphetamine	97
Ecstasy	80
Solvents	1,070
Opiates (mainly heroin and methadone)	2,395

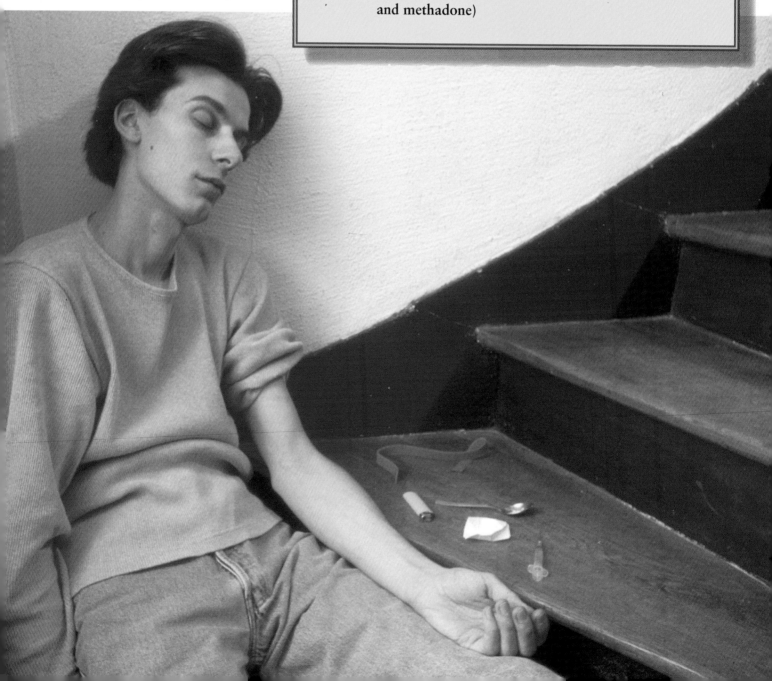

RISKS

However, taking any drug is always a gamble. You cannot tell what is in them or how you will react. Combining different drugs, especially on top of drinking alcohol, is particularly risky. The sad fact is that taking illegal drugs does kill a significant number of people every year.

One of the most dangerous drug activities is abusing solvents like glue or aerosols. The risk of suffocation or choking on vomit is high, as is the chance of sudden heart failure. Heroin and crack cocaine can kill through overdose, particularly if the drug is unexpectedly pure. Ecstasy has led to a significant number of deaths in the UK, by encouraging overheating and dehydration in users. Some users have died by drinking too much water to compensate.

DRUG-RELATED DEATHS

However, not all deaths are related directly to the drug. Like alcohol, many illegal drugs kill by increasing the risk of accidents. Driving under the effect of illegal drugs is particularly foolish, and may harm others as well as yourself.

Becoming dependent on drugs can have other consequences. Drugs are very expensive and can lead to financial problems. You can also lose your friends or even your job if the effects of taking drugs starts to alter your behaviour or your ability to function normally.

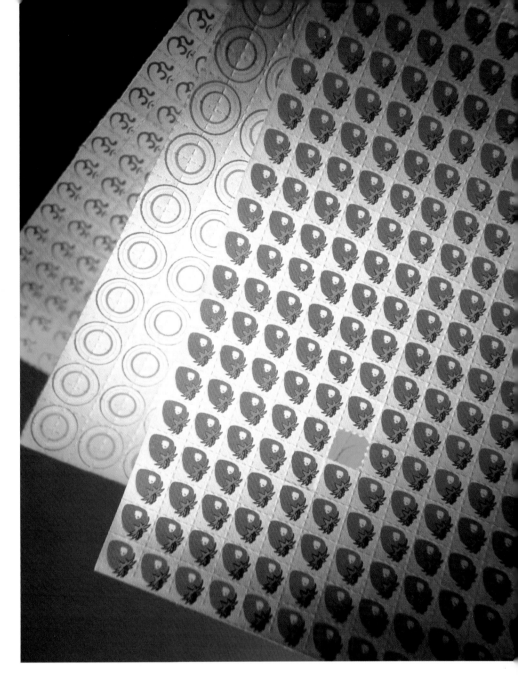

LSD is made in the form of tablets and as sheets of blotting paper that are cut into squares and impregnated with the drug. LSD, or 'acid', is illegal in most countries but is widely used as a recreational drug.

HALLUCINATIONS

Some drugs like LSD, magic mushrooms or even cannabis can cause hallucinations, where you see, hear or feel things that aren't really happening. They can be very frightening. Many drugs cause panic attacks, which can be very alarming, even leading people to believe that they are dying. This is particularly likely if someone is anxious or worried about the drug's effects.

MEDICINAL DRUGS

HOW DO MEDICINAL DRUGS AFFECT ME?

Not so long ago, the only drugs or medicines available for people were substances extracted from plants and sometimes animals. Indeed, in some countries like China, the use of herbs and other plants is still a popular way of treating the sick.

Despite dramatic leaps in medical technology, some illnesses, such as the common cold and flu, still have no cure.

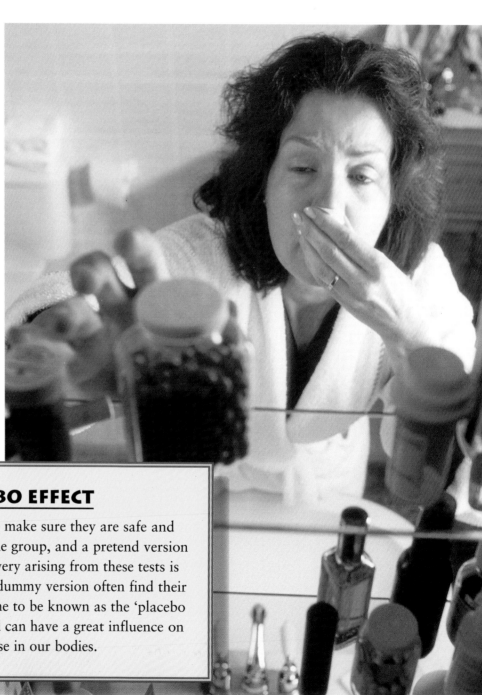

THE PLACEBO EFFECT

New drugs are always tested to make sure they are safe and effective, by giving the drug to one group, and a pretend version to another. An interesting discovery arising from these tests is that even those people given the dummy version often find their symptoms improve. This has come to be known as the 'placebo effect' and is proof that the mind can have a great influence on the course of disease in our bodies.

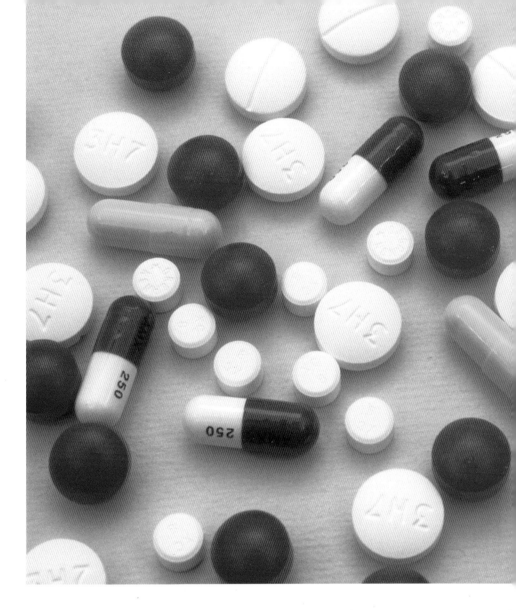

DEVELOPING DRUGS

In much of the world, however, modern medicine relies heavily on drugs created in the laboratory, manufactured through various chemical processes. There are drugs for every type of illness and disorder, and thousands more are developed every year.

HOW DO THEY WORK?

While the exact workings of some drugs are poorly understood, most work either by replacing deficient chemicals in the body, interfering with the ways in which cells function, or by combating infectious diseases and bacteria. Some drugs work very rapidly to relieve symptoms of disease; others can take months to have any effect.

SIDE-EFFECTS

All drugs, however, have unwanted as well as desired effects on the body, called side-effects. When you take a drug, it travels to all parts of your body, and may work on parts other than those affected by the illness or disease. Some people are more vulnerable to side-effects than others, and may even stop taking a drug because of them.

COMMON DRUGS AND SIDE-EFFECTS

DRUG	USE	SIDE EFFECTS
Fluoxetine (Prozac)	Antidepressant	Headache, diarrhoea, anxiety
Aspirin	Painkiller	Indigestion
Morphine	Painkiller	Drowsiness, nausea, constipation
Ranitidine (Zantac)	Anti-ulcer drug	Headache
Antibiotics	Anti-infection drug	Diarrhoea, rash

DRUGS IN SPORT

Drug	Why taken	Is it banned?	Why?
Anabolic Steroids	To build muscle bulk	Yes	Gives users an unfair advantage and is associated with many health problems
Caffeine	To stimulate the body	Only in very large quantities	
Cocaine	To stimulate the body	Yes	Many health risks
Morphine	To reduce or remove pain	Yes	Can cover up underlying fitness problems

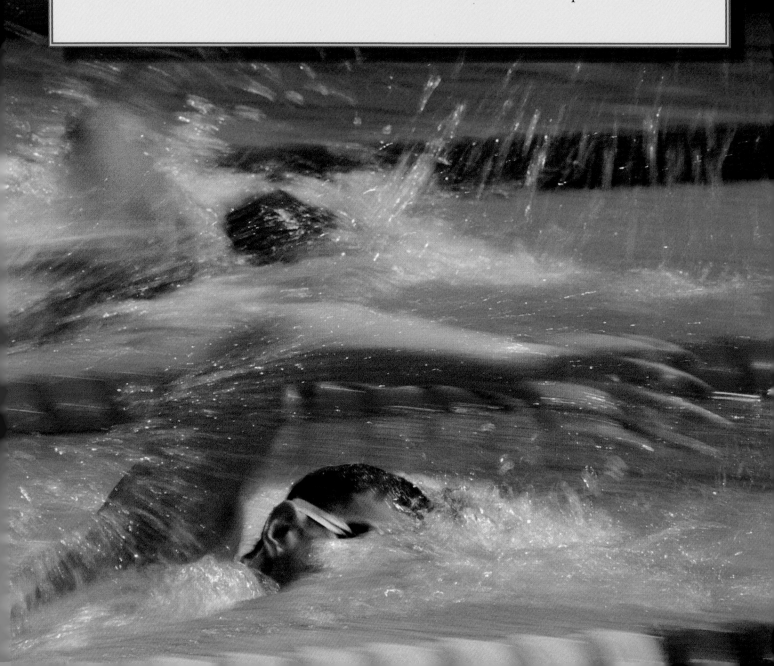

ABUSING MEDICINAL DRUGS

Medical drugs can be just as powerful as illegal drugs like heroin or cocaine, and just as dangerous if not used properly. Sometimes medical drugs are deliberately abused; the sleeping pill Temazepam is sometimes sold on the street. Melting down these capsules and injecting them into the bloodstream can cause blockages, sometimes leading to limb amputations or even death.

ADVERSE REACTIONS

More often, however, medicinal drugs cause accidental harm. All drugs are chemicals, and can have a toxic effect on the body. Some people have an adverse reaction to a drug they need, and in extreme cases this can kill. Sometimes one drug may react with another that a person is taking, producing powerful and unwanted results.

MIXING DRUGS

Other drugs such as alcohol, can interfere with certain medications like some antidepressants, sedatives and antibiotics. Sometimes drugs like antihistamines, used to treat allergies, can make users very drowsy, and increase the chances of car or industrial accidents.

Anabolic steroids improve performance by stimulating muscle and bone growth.

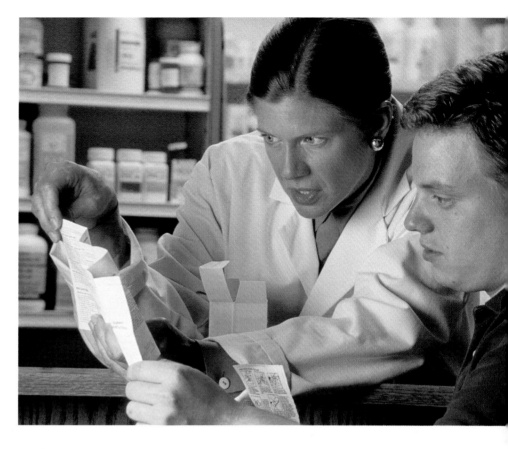

DANGERS OF MEDICINAL DRUGS

Drugs can be dangerous in different situations. Young children should never take the painkiller aspirin as sometimes it can cause a potentially fatal condition called Reye's Syndrome. Pregnant women must avoid drugs which could damage their unborn baby. In the 1960s, for instance, many children were born handicapped because their mothers were prescribed the anti-sickness drug Thalidomide during pregnancy.

Sometimes people become addicted to medicinal drugs. For many years, doctors prescribed tranquillizers, used to treat anxiety, not realizing that by taking them that their patients were becoming addicted to them.

It is very important that people follow the instructions precisely when taking medicinal drugs. Otherwise they may experience adverse reactions.

CANCER CURE

Occasionally the toxic effects of a drug are deliberate. The common cancer treatment, chemotherapy, works by poisoning the cells in the body. The hope is that the healthy ones will recover, while the cancerous cells die. Because of this toxicity, chemotherapy is often an unpleasant treatment to undergo.

BEING SENSIBLE

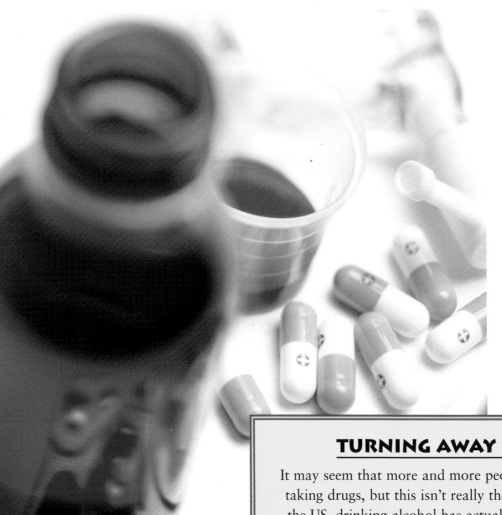

Few people would suggest that we ban alcohol completely. Indeed many people depend on it for their jobs, and alcohols such as wine are appreciated by millions of people across the world without posing a great risk to their health. Indeed, small amounts of alcohol have been shown to actually lower the risk of heart disease in older men.

AVOIDING THE RISKS

Other drugs, however, such as tobacco and illegal drugs, are always best avoided. No one will claim that taking them is likely to kill you – at least, not immediately.

TURNING AWAY FROM DRUGS

It may seem that more and more people are smoking, drinking and taking drugs, but this isn't really the case. In Western Europe and the US, drinking alcohol has actually decreased over the last 100 years. In the UK smoking has reduced from 50 per cent of adults smoking in 1972 to around 30 per cent today. Even fears that we're in the grip of an escalating drug crisis could be based on a myth; the largest UK survey of drug misuse shows that drug taking is not part of normal behaviour for the vast majority of young people.

Nearly all drugs are potentially dangerous if taken irresponsibly – even cold and flu remedies.

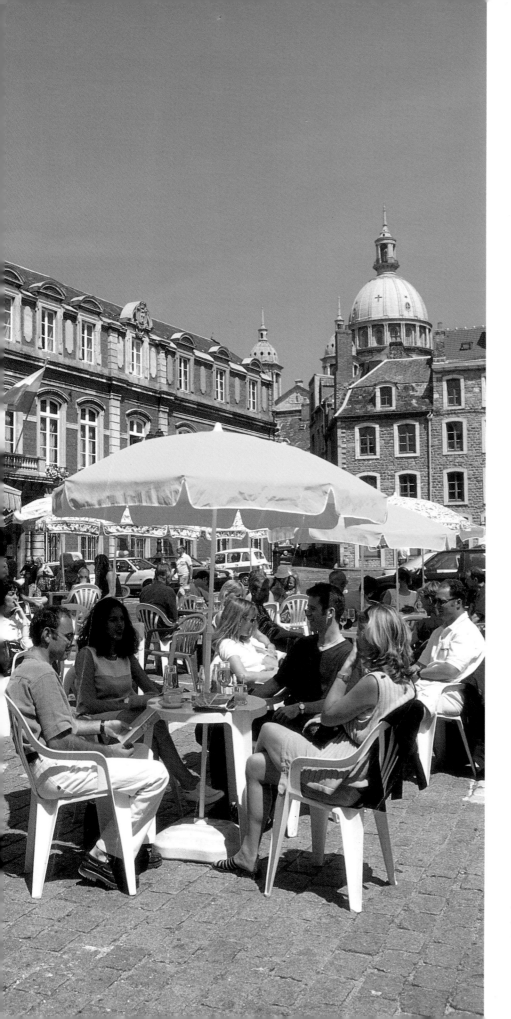

But all of them are bad for your health in one way or another, and can have serious consequences for you physically and mentally. Many of these consequences only show up later in life; unfortunately by then it is often too late to do anything about them.

LIFE-SAVING DRUGS

Medicines, on the other hand, save thousands of lives every year. We are lucky to be living at a time when we have chemicals to help cure and control the diseases that have plagued mankind for thousands of years. Antibiotics can cure infections that would have killed less than a century ago.

But all drugs, even medicines, have to be used sensibly. Too many antibiotics, for instance, can actually provoke disease, by encouraging the bacteria that cause them to mutate. Those people who avoid harmful drugs and treat medicines with respect stand to gain the most from what these modern chemicals can offer.

With so many medicines available to us today, modern life has the potential to be full and active. To realize this potential, people must have a sensible approach to drugs and alcohol.

GLOSSARY

Amputation When a limb is cut off for a medical reason.

Antacids Medicine taken for certain stomach upsets.

Apathy A feeling of not caring about things.

Arteries The main blood carrying tubes in your body.

Bacteria Tiny organisms that sometimes cause diseases.

Central nervous system The brain and the spinal cord system controlling the body's working and reactions.

Convulsion When someone shakes, as in a fit.

Craving When you feel a desperate wish to have something.

Dehydration When your body loses too much water.

Dependence When somebody is unable to live and cope without taking a particular drug.

Depression A feeling of sadness over a period of time.

Dilate To widen or expand.

Fermentation A chemical reaction that breaks down a molecule, such as when yeast breaks down sugar into alcohol.

Genetic Tendencies or conditions which are inherited from your parents.

Hallucinations Visions of something that isn't actually there.

Hepatitis A disease of the liver.

Incontinence An inability to control the bladder or bowels, often brought on by excessive alcohol intake.

Immune system The system that the body relies on to defend itself from infection.

Impregnate To saturate or soak an item with something, such as a liquid.

Inhale To breath and draw air or other gases into the lungs.

Mineral A substance that is from neither an animal or plant.

Muslim A person who believes and follows the Islamic religion.

Paranoia A feeling that other people are 'out to get you'.

Persecution When someone is hounded and mistreated.

Placebo Something, such as a drug, that is ineffective but is given to someone to make them think that they are being treated.

Plantation An estate where huge crops, such as tobacco, rubber and bananas, are grown for export to other countries.

Psychological Something that relates to your mind or feelings.

Schizophrenia A mental illness that results in people withdrawing from society and hallucinating.

'Snort' To inhale something, such as a drug, through the nose.

Steroids Drugs, such as anabolic steroids, that can be used to improve sporting performance by building up muscle.

Stimulant Something that excites or speeds up the workings of the mind or body.

Ulcer A sore area on the inside or outside of your body.

Unit of alcohol The amount of alcohol used to stimulate a certain effect.

Vapour When a liquid evaporates it forms particles of moisture which are called vapour.

Vial A small bottle used to contain liquids.

Vitamin An element that is essential in small quantities for providing nutrition to the body.

Withdrawal The period that a drug-user goes through after giving up using drugs. Usually associated with physical and mental side effects.

FURTHER INFORMATION

FURTHER READING

We're Talking About Alcohol by Jenny Bryan (Wayland, 1995)
We're Talking About Smoking by Karen Bryant-Mole (Wayland, 1997)
Life Files: Drugs by Julian Cohen (Evans Brothers, 1998)
Alcohol by Emma Haughton (Wayland, 1998)
Drugs by Adrian King (Wayland, 1997)
Talking Points: Mental Illness by Vanora Leigh (Wayland, 1999)
Talking Points: Family Violence by Ronda Armitage (Wayland, 1999)
Know About Smoking by Margaret O'Hyde (Walker and Co, 1997)
Drinking Alcohol by Steve Myers and Pete Sanders (Franklin Watts, 1996)
What Do You Know About Aids? by Pete Sanders and Steve Myers (Franklin Watts, 1996)
What Do You Know About Drugs? by Pete Sanders and Steve Myers (Franklin Watts, 1996)
What Do You Know About Smoking? by Pete Sanders and Steve Myers (Franklin Watts, 1994)
Let's Talk About Smoking by Elizabeth Weitzman and Rudolf Steiner (Powerkids Press, 1998)

FINDING OUT MORE

Health Education Authority,
Trevelyan House,
30 Great Peter Street,
London SW1P 2HW
Tel: 0207 413 1888
www.hea.org.uk

Alcohol Concern,
Waterbridge House,
32–36 Loman Street,
London SE1 0EE
Tel: 0207 928 7377
www.alcoholconcern.org.uk

Alcoholics Anonymous,
PO Box 1,
Stonebow House,
Stonebow,
York YO1 2NJ
Tel: 01904 644026

Brook Advisory Centres
(throughout UK)
Details on contraception clinics:
0800 0185 023

ChildLine,
Freepost 1111,
London N1 0BR
Freephone: 0800 1111
Website: www.childline.org.uk

Depression Alliance,
35, Westminster Bridge Road,
London SE1 7JB
Tel: 0207 633 0557

Scotland: 0131 467 3050
Wales 01222 611674
Website: www.gn.apc.org/da/

Drinkline Youth (For Confidential, advice about drinking)
0345 230202

Ash – Action on Smoking and Health,
16 Fitzhardinge Street,
London W1H 9PL
Tel: 0207 224 0743
www.ash.co.uk

INDEX